W9-AVA-577

Can I tell you about ME/Chronic Fatigue Syndrome?

Can I tell you about...?

The "Can I tell you about...?" series offers simple introductions to a range of limiting conditions. Friendly characters invite readers to learn about their experiences of living with a particular condition and how they would like to be helped and supported. These books serve as excellent starting points for family and classroom discussions.

Other subjects covered in the "Can I tell you about...?" series

ADHD

Adoption

Asperger Syndrome

Asthma

Cerebral Palsy

Dementia

Dyslexia

Epilepsy

OCD

Parkinson's Disease

Selective Mutism

Stammering/Stuttering

Tourette Syndrome

Can I tell you about ME/ Chronic Fatigue Syndrome?

A guide for friends, family and professionals

JACQUELINE RAYNER

Illustrated by Jason Lythgoe-Hay

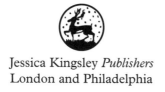

Jessica Kingsley *Publishers*
London and Philadelphia

First published in 2014
by Jessica Kingsley Publishers
73 Collier Street
London N1 9BE, UK
and
400 Market Street, Suite 400
Philadelphia, PA 19106, USA

www.jkp.com

Copyright © Jacqueline Rayner 2014
Illustrations copyright © Jason Lythgoe-Hay 2014

All rights reserved. No part of this publication may be reproduced in
any material form (including photocopying or storing it in any medium
by electronic means and whether or not transiently or incidentally to
some other use of this publication) without the written permission of the
copyright owner except in accordance with the provisions of the Copyright,
Designs and Patents Act 1988 or under the terms of a licence issued by the
Copyright Licensing Agency Ltd, Saffron House, 6–10 Kirby Street, London
EC1N 8TS. Applications for the copyright owner's written permission to
reproduce any part of this publication should be addressed to the publisher.

Warning: The doing of an unauthorised act in relation to a copyright work
may result in both a civil claim for damages and criminal prosecution.

Library of Congress Cataloging in Publication Data
Rayner, Jacqueline.
Can I tell you about ME/chronic fatigue syndrome? :
a guide for friends, family and professionals /
Jacqueline Rayner ; illustrated by Jason Lythgoe-Hay.
pages cm. -- (Can I tell you about...?)
ISBN 978-1-84905-452-2 (alk. paper)
1. Chronic fatigue syndrome--Juvenile literature. I. Lythgoe-
Hay, Jason, illustrator. II. Title. III. Title: Can
I tell you about myalgic encephalomyelitis, chronic fatigue syndrome?
RB150.F37.R39 2014
616'.044--dc23
2013047817

British Library Cataloguing in Publication Data
A CIP catalogue record for this book is available from the British Library

ISBN 978 1 84905 452 2
eISBN 978 0 85700 826 8

Printed and bound in Great Britain by Bell and Bain Ltd, Glasgow

Acknowledgements

Thanks to Mum, Dad and Helen, Debbie and Graham Brent, India Crewe, Roger Dilley, Jan Farrow, Emma Summers, Mrs Bird from Class 4, Jason the illustrator extraordinaire, the amazing people at Invest in ME and the fabulous fundraisers of Let's Do It for ME! (http:// ldifme.org), and of course my wonderful children and my husband Nick.

Contents

Introduction

There are lots of books that deal with the medical side of ME, and lots that offer tips for improving symptoms or coping with illness. That's not what this book does. Although it is hoped that it will be informative about the disease, its main aim is to show what life can be like if someone in a family has ME.

No two people's illnesses are ever the same, and that's especially true of ME. People with ME may have all sorts of different symptoms. They may have it very mildly and be able to work and go out, or they may be so ill that they are unable to get out of bed and have to be fed through a tube.

Because this book is based on the experience of one family, it may not all be relevant to every sufferer or their family, but we hope there will be something in it for everyone.

Life can be difficult for children who have an ill parent. One of the aims of this book is to help those children (and their friends and teachers) gain a clearer understanding of ME.

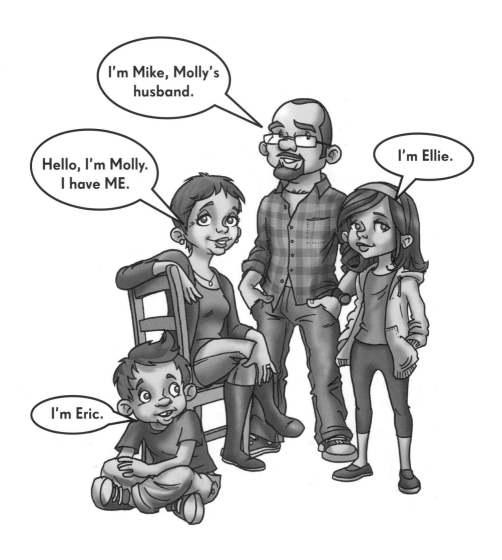

"On the outside, our family might look just like many other families, but ME/CFS makes things different for us. We'd like to tell you about it."

Molly says:

"Most illnesses are quite easy to explain. ME isn't! Even deciding what to call the illness is complicated – we'll talk more about that on p.45. But for now, you just need to know that this book is for you if a doctor has said that you (or someone you know) has ME (myalgic encephalomyelitis), CFS (chronic fatigue syndrome), PVFS (post-viral fatigue syndrome) or ME/CFS. We're going to be using the term PWME (person/people with ME) to mean someone who has any of those.

ME is an illness that affects your body and your brain, especially the nervous system (your brain, spinal cord and nerves) and the immune system (the bits that prevent or fight disease).

People are still trying to find out what causes it – doctors have all sorts of ideas, and sometimes even argue about who is right. For some people, the illness comes on slowly and it might be years before the doctors decide what's wrong with them (this is 'gradual onset ME'). It wasn't like that for me – I became ill with glandular fever (sometimes called 'mono') when I was young and just never really got better, even when the virus had gone away. (This is 'sudden onset ME', which usually has a trigger such as a virus.) The virus must have caused some damage that my body can't fix, but until doctors find out exactly what the damage is, they can't make me better."

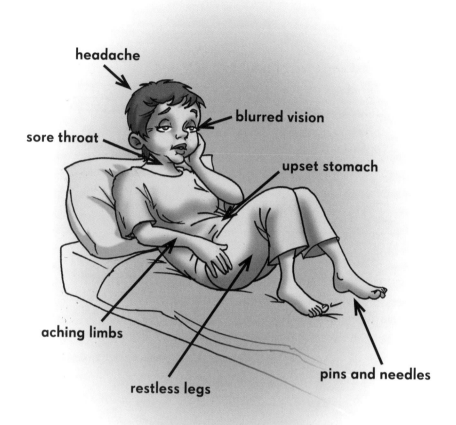

"There are lots of things that can go wrong
with your body when you have ME."

Molly says:

"PWME have all sorts of different symptoms. (A symptom is something that happens to your body because of your illness.) Some of the most common problems include: muscle/joint pain; 'cognitive dysfunction' (for example, memory or concentration problems); fainting or dizziness; sore throat and 'flu-like' feelings; headaches; sleep problems; digestive problems (for example, feeling sick or having stomach pains), or seizures (for example falling unconscious or limbs jerking).

Everyone who has ME has one particular symptom, though: PEM (post-exertional malaise, also called post-exertional neuroimmune exhaustion or PENE). This is when a PWME becomes very unwell following any form of exertion (not just physical activities but mental too). Sometimes the PEM doesn't appear until a day or two after the activity that caused it. I'll explain more about this later.

When I was first ill, my main symptoms were fatigue plus a very sore throat when I'd done too much (I used to describe it as like having a golf ball covered in razor blades stuck in my throat). Now new symptoms pop up all the time, most recently shooting pains in different parts of my body and 'pins and needles' in my legs and feet. Having ME is a bit like a lucky dip – you never know what symptom you'll wake up with next! (Maybe that should be an *unlucky* dip...)"

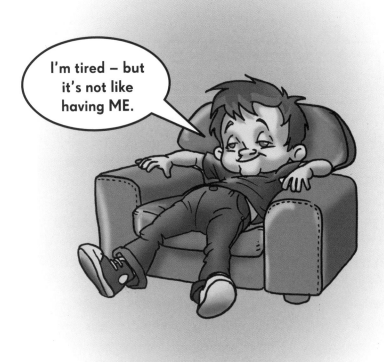

"ME 'fatigue' isn't like normal tiredness."

Eric says:

"A lot of people think 'fatigue' just means tired. You know what being tired feels like, right? It's how you feel when you've had a really busy day. You just want to sit down and watch the telly, or maybe go straight to bed for a sleep. Mum says the fatigue you get with ME isn't like that. Your body might be so tired you can't move it at all, even if you try really hard. Your brain might get really tired too, and you find it hard to understand things – people with ME call this 'brain fog'. The tiredness you get with ME is more like how you feel if you have flu – imagine having flu every single day!"

Molly says:

"You'd think I wouldn't have any problems sleeping, but no! A lot of PWME suffer from insomnia (that's when it's hard to fall asleep or to stay asleep). Bedtime can turn into a nightmare – a waking nightmare! Mind you, some PWME have the opposite problem – they sleep and sleep and sleep and are only awake for a few hours in a day. If you're a PWME who sleeps a lot, or you take medicine that helps you sleep, it might seem like you're getting all the rest you need. Unfortunately, that's not the case. PWME's sleep can be very restless and full of vivid dreams, and it doesn't make them feel refreshed afterwards."

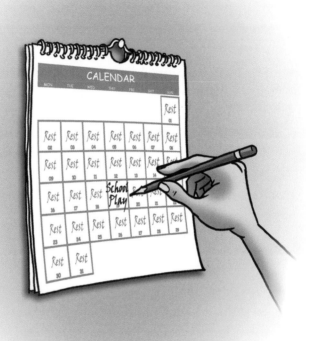

"It can be hard to plan things
when you have ME."

Ellie says:

"One weird thing is that Mum never knows when the fatigue will hit. Imagine you went on a very long walk. You might start to get tired after you'd been walking for a while, and by the time you got home you might be really worn out. Things don't follow so simply for Mum. She might be walking along feeling OK when suddenly her body gives up and she can't walk another step. Or she might do the whole walk and feel OK, but then the next day or the day after that she will feel really ill and might have to stay in bed for a week.

That means it's really hard to plan things when your mum has ME. If Mum knows there's something important coming up, like one of us having a birthday or a parents' evening at school, she'll try to spend several days before it resting, and will make sure she doesn't have lots of things to do in the days after it so she can recover. This doesn't always work, though."

Molly says:

"I try not to show how upset I am when I miss something, because I don't want to spoil it for everyone else. But I don't want the children to think I don't care about being with them or going to something they've worked hard on, like a school play. It's tough getting the balance right."

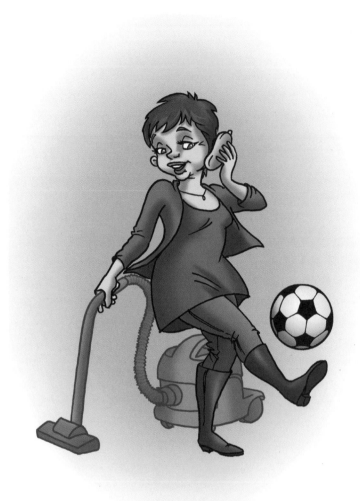

"When I have a good day, I want to do
everything – but it's not a good idea."

Molly says:

"ME is a 'fluctuating condition'. That means the illness can change from day to day – or even from hour to hour. I have 'good days' and 'bad days'. On bad days I might not even be able to get out of bed. On good days, I might be able to go shopping or go to the cinema.

Something that is very important when you have ME is *pacing*. Pacing means not pushing your body too far – you have to make sure you stop an activity *before* it becomes too demanding for you. It's the best way of coping with ME, but it's very difficult, especially if you have children.

There are so many things I want to do, from playing with my children to going shopping to tidying the house. When I have a good day, it's hard not to try to do all of them! Sometimes I don't judge things very well. I think I can manage something – perhaps going shopping or doing some gardening – but it turns out it's too much for me. Having support from my family really helps. Sometimes they can see when I need to slow down better than I can myself."

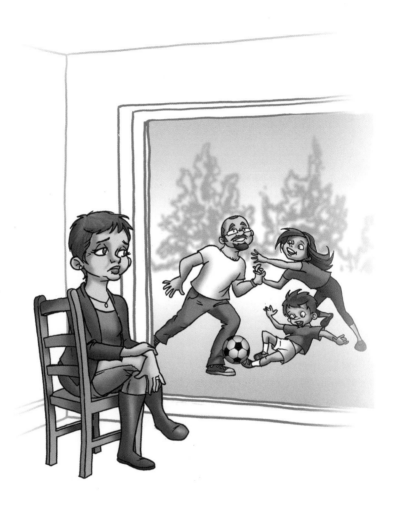

"It's hard for Mum when she can't join in our games, but it's more important for her to rest."

Eric says:

"Mum's bad days are rotten for everyone, but we have to be careful on Mum's good days too. Mum really hates not being able to do stuff with us, and so sometimes when she feels a bit better she tries to make up for that by doing as much as she can. The trouble is, that can make her *really* ill. So we try to make sure that anything we do won't tire her out too much – we might have to be the grown-up and tell Mum she can't play football with us, even if she wants to and we want her to too!"

Molly says:

"Physical activity is difficult for me – but admitting I needed help was almost as difficult.

These days, I use a walking stick and a wheelchair and a mobility scooter. I also have other things that help me, like a shower seat and handrails. But it took me a long time to come to terms with needing them. One reason was that it made me feel like I was giving in to my illness – like ME and I were having a fight about who was in charge, and I was letting ME win. But as well as that, it made me feel guilty. I felt that things like wheelchairs were for people who couldn't walk at all, not people like me who could manage to walk a little bit, even if it was difficult."

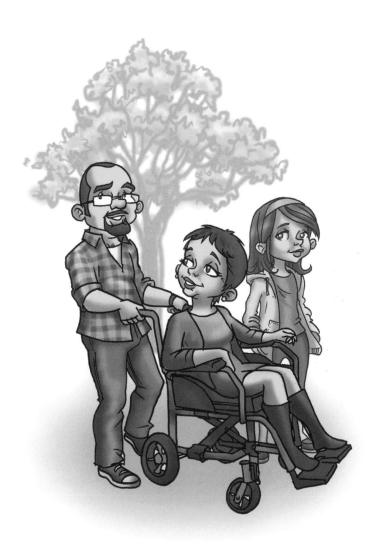

"Using aids doesn't mean you've given in to your illness – it means you've found a way of coping."

Molly says:

"Things got much easier for me after I accepted that I needed help. Having a walking stick doesn't just help me hobble about when I have low energy, it also gives me confidence that I have support if I suddenly get weak or dizzy. I'm no longer always left at home when my family go out – if I'm well enough to leave the house, someone can push me in my wheelchair. On top of that, if I use my wheelchair on an outing *even when I'm well enough to walk*, it means I might not get too ill later on.

I've had some funny looks from people who don't know me. They might see a person who is using a walking stick, but appears to be able to walk easily. They might see a person who gets out of their wheelchair and walks about, no problem at all. I can understand why they think it's odd, but I also know that I'm doing the right thing for my health and my family."

Ellie says:

"Sometimes people say rude things about Mum, because she uses a wheelchair or a walking stick. They think she's pretending, or that she's doing it to get sympathy – or that she's just lazy. Sometimes we get teased too, and called names, just because our mum's ill. We know we have to ignore things like that and try not to get upset. *We* know our mum isn't lazy or pretending, and that's what's important."

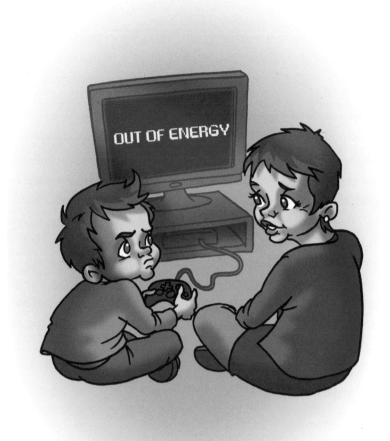

"Mum says ME is a bit like a video game where you keep running out of energy."

Eric says:

"I love video games, but it's really annoying when you run out of energy or lives and you can't keep playing, or are sent right back to the beginning. Sometimes you have to save up points for ages to get a particular ability or item. Mum says ME is a bit like that. This is how she explained it to us:

Imagine a video game: 'Normal Life'.

Each player starts with a certain amount of energy – perhaps 1000 points. During the course of a day they spend these points on activities.

Every activity has an energy price tag:

Getting out of bed: 1pt

Walking to bathroom: 1pt

Having a shower: 3pt

Washing your hair: 3pt

Getting dressed: 2pt

Going downstairs: 3pt

Walking to kitchen: 1pt

Filling kettle: 2pt

Making a cup of tea: 1pt

Writing an essay: 15pt

Reading a book: 3pt"

Molly says:

"At the end of the day, the player probably still has a few points left. Overnight, their energy points are topped up, so they start the next day with a full energy store. Sometimes, if they don't sleep very well or a bug gets in the system, the energy store doesn't fill right up overnight, but once the bug is fixed it returns to normal.

A player who has ME starts off each day with a much smaller energy store – perhaps between one and 100 points. The most severe sufferers may have zero points.

Imagine a housebound sufferer who starts a day with ten energy points. They probably can't top up their energy store during the day (although having a nap *might* give them back one or two points), so they have to be very careful in deciding what to spend their points on. For example, if they choose to have a shower and wash their hair, it means they will not have enough points left to go downstairs and make themselves a cup of tea.

The mechanism that refills the energy store overnight doesn't work properly in PWME, so they never know how many points they will have the next morning. It might be 50 – or it might be five."

Molly says:

"A player with ME who knows they will need a certain amount of points for an activity in the future has to try to save up their energy. If a friend is visiting in the afternoon, the player has to spend as few points as possible in the morning. If the player is planning a trip to the cinema at the weekend, they may have to save their points for days – they can only hope that each night will add enough points so they have enough by the time they're needed.

Sometimes, the game allows players to buy extra energy points. This might mean they're able to carry out an activity that costs more than their daily energy allowance. The trouble is, each extra energy point might cost three or four energy points to buy, and sooner or later the player will have to pay up. So buying some extra energy to spend on a Saturday might mean the PWME won't have any more energy points for a week.

It's very difficult to win at this game. Players just have to try to keep going as long as possible."

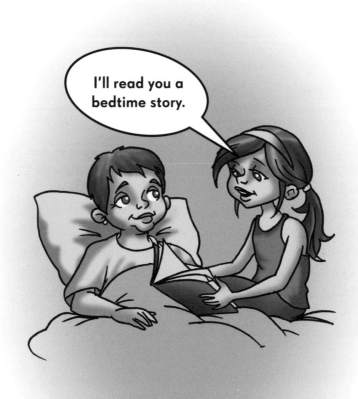

"Sometimes it's hard to tell who's the grown-up in the family."

Molly says:

"When I was little, my mum and dad looked after me. I thought that when I grew up and became a parent, I would look after my children. I also thought that my parents wouldn't have to look after me any longer. I was wrong!

ME often means losing your independence, and this can be difficult.

I'm one of the lucky ones because I have family who are willing to look after me and help look after my children. Some PWME have carers arranged privately or through social services. Some PWME don't get the help they need and have to struggle on the best they can.

Having carers can be difficult. It's not very nice having a stranger wash you or help you use the toilet. If family help you, you might feel guilty that they have to give up their free time.

One symptom of ME is 'emotional lability'. This means you get mood swings, or you may get very upset about something unimportant. You might cry for no real reason, or because of something trivial. You might get irritated very easily. Of course, this sort of thing doesn't just happen to a PWME – but it's helpful if your friends and family understand that your reactions to things might be a bit over the top and you can't help it.

I hate my children seeing me get upset. I'm supposed to be the grown-up, yet they often end up comforting me instead of the other way around."

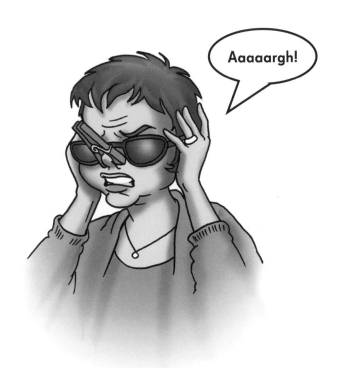

"Sound, light and smell can hurt someone who has ME."

Ellie says:

"Sometimes PWME feel like their senses have been turned up to maximum! Even really ordinary things can make them feel ill. Mum doesn't like going to the cinema because it's very loud and the screen is very bright, and the movement on the screen makes her feel a bit sick and dizzy.

We have to be careful at home too, if Mum's feeling poorly. Noises can hurt her ears, so we try not to shout and we don't play our music too loudly. Bright lights might hurt her eyes, so sometimes she has to have the curtains drawn even in the daytime. Even strong smells can make Mum feel ill – Dad mustn't wear any aftershave when she's having a bad day!"

Molly says:

"I'm lucky because these things only upset me on my worst days. Some people who have ME badly feel like this all the time. They just stay in bed with the curtains closed and no lights on, and it has to be totally quiet. Just having people come in to their room might cause them pain. It's hard to imagine what it must be like to live your whole life in bed with nothing to do and not even any company, but people who are that ill don't have any choice."

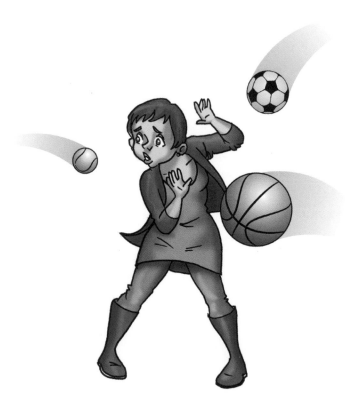

"Too many things happening at once can overload your senses."

Molly says:

"Sounds and lights and smells only cause problems for me occasionally, but there are other things connected with the senses that affect me much more often. It's very easy to make me jump, just by coming into a room or speaking when I wasn't expecting it. It's also very easy for my senses to become overwhelmed; for example, if two people are talking to me at once, I can't concentrate on what either of them is saying and it can make me feel quite panicky. Sometimes this happens if only one person is talking to me but the television is on or there's traffic noise coming from outside – I can't filter out the extra signals.

Imagine someone gently throwing a ball to you. You see it coming and can catch it easily. Now imagine being pelted by lots of balls all being thrown – hard – at the same time. You probably won't be able to catch any of them, or even take in the shape or colour of all the different balls. You might also feel under attack. That's a bit what it can be like for a PWME when there are lots of things going on at once. We call it 'sensory overload'."

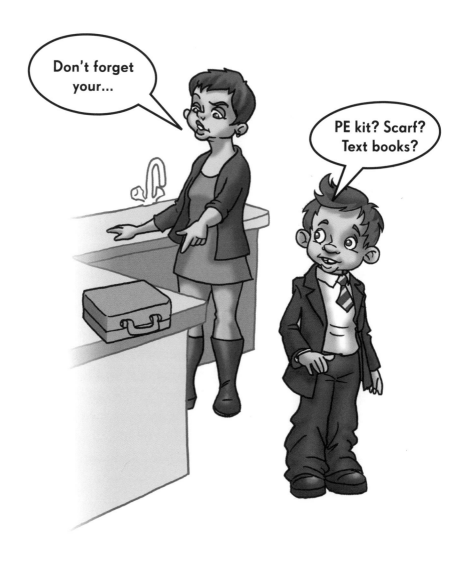

"Sometimes Mum can't remember the word she needs to use."

Eric says:

"Sometimes when Mum's in the middle of talking she can't think of the word she needs. It might be a really easy word, such as 'fridge' or 'door'! She calls this 'losing words', and it happens when something in her brain stops her making a connection. It can be awkward if she's talking to someone who doesn't know her well or doesn't really understand about her illness."

Molly says:

"Forgetting words is one of the reasons that I don't really like talking on the telephone, except to close friends or family. If I have to make a phone call I usually make notes of important points beforehand. Short-term memory is another big problem for PWME, so I write things down a *lot*.

There is another reason I don't like talking on the telephone, though. It's because it requires me to be 'on'. What exactly is being 'on'? Well, it's one of the differences between your private and your public face. Most people will switch on – for a conversation, or when paying for something in a shop, or even writing an email – and they might not even realise they're doing it. The reason that people with ME can be strongly aware of being 'on' is because it uses up energy.

Being 'on' is a natural part of being with other people, even close friends. It's why social occasions can be exhausting for PWME, even if they never move from their chair!"

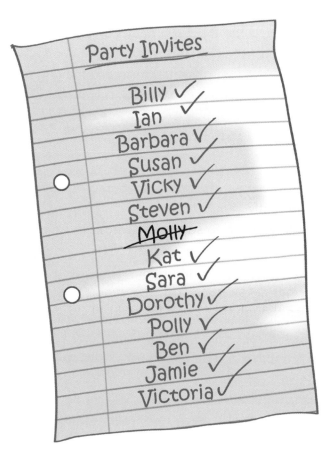

"It's not unusual for PWME to lose friends."

Molly says:

"Some people with mild ME have full-time jobs. The trouble is, they might be using up nearly all their 'energy points' to do their job. That means they have to say no to things like drinks after work or even just going out for lunch. Things can get awkward because people think you're unfriendly – especially because some PWME don't want to tell anyone they're ill, in case they are treated differently.

PWME often have to say no to invitations from friends too, and it's not unusual for PWME to lose friends who don't understand their situation.

Sometimes my friends ask if they should invite me to things, even though they know I'll probably be too ill to go. Does it look like they don't understand that I'm ill, or will it upset me to know I'm missing out on all the fun? But if they don't send me an invite, will I be hurt at being missed out?

Other PWME might have a different opinion to me, but I like it when I'm still included in invitations. It's extra nice if the person sending the invitation shows that they understand my situation, though. So if an invitation says something like, 'I know it'll probably be too difficult for you to come, but it would be lovely if you could' or 'Please don't worry about replying if you can't come, I know it uses up your energy', it makes a big difference."

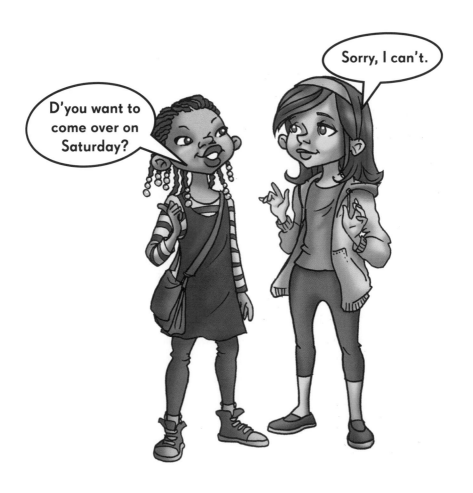

"Everyone's social life suffers when someone in the family has ME."

Ellie says:

"Mum doesn't get to see her friends very much, but sometimes we don't get to see our friends either. People with ME can drive, but Mum decided to stop driving when her illness got worse because she didn't feel safe any more – if she suddenly got dizzy or her legs became weak she might have an accident. Most of the time she's not even well enough to walk to the bus stop. That means she can't take us to play dates. Our friends can't come over to play at our house very often either; it'd be too much for Mum.

If Mum's friends visit, she's usually so pleased to see them that she doesn't care how much energy it uses up! Unexpected visitors can be awkward, though, because if Mum hasn't prepared for a visit, she has to use up energy that she might have been saving for something else, or try to buy extra energy that she'll need to pay back later (see p.27).

Mum worries that people will think us rude because we say no to going out and don't invite people to our house very much. *We* worry that our friends will think we don't like them and will get upset. They might stop inviting us to their birthday parties, and maybe even not want to be our friends any more. If people understood more about what it's like when someone in your family has ME, we wouldn't worry so much about losing friends. "

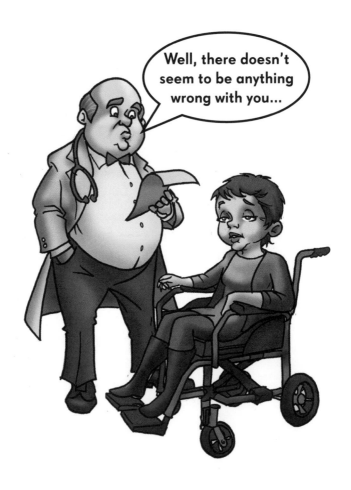

"Proving you're ill can be a problem."

Molly says:

"I try to think positively most of the time. It's not always easy, though. I didn't imagine my life would be like this. Sometimes I remember what I used to be like, what I used to be able to do, and I feel very miserable. It's not unusual to be depressed if you have ME – but that doesn't mean that ME is a kind of depression.

It can also be depressing (and frustrating) when you're a PWME if you have to spend a lot of time convincing people that you're physically ill. There are lots of studies that show all sorts of things that are going wrong in the bodies of PWME (you can find out more by following the links on pp.59–61), but our biggest problem is that there isn't yet a single test doctors can do to show if someone has ME or not.

In the UK (and some other countries), there are official lists of the treatments and tests for each illness. Unfortunately, most of the tests and treatments that have been found to work for PWME aren't yet on the lists. This means that even doctors who understand about ME can't always do anything to help you.

Some doctors think that ME is just in people's minds. They haven't looked – or don't want to look – at all the evidence that shows it isn't. This can be very upsetting for patients. Feeling that no one can help, or even wants to, is another reason why people with this illness can feel pretty low."

Molly says:

"Because ME isn't understood very well, even by doctors, it can carry a stigma – that's when other people think badly of you. No one wants to be thought of as a hypochondriac (someone who makes a big fuss about being ill although there's nothing wrong with them). No one wants to be seen as lazy, or as someone who's only pretending to be ill. That's why some people with ME don't tell others that they're ill. I didn't for ages, until I got too poorly to hide my illness all the time.

Here are some of the things that are sometimes said about ME:

- 'It's mind over matter. If you have a positive attitude, you'll stop being ill.' WRONG!

- 'All you need to do is exercise.' WRONG!

- 'It's burn-out – you just need to rest for a bit and you'll be OK.' WRONG!

- 'It's all in your head. Try telling yourself you're not ill.' WRONG!

- 'You're just scared of exerting yourself.' WRONG!

Some of these things are not just wrong, they could be harmful. For example, for most people, exercise makes them healthier – for PWME, it makes them worse! A person with mild ME who tries to make themselves better by exercising could easily end up with severe ME."

"Many PWME also regularly hear the same sort of things from (well-meaning) friends:

- 'I read about a course you can do that cures ME.'

- 'I heard that exercise and counselling cure ME.'

- 'Here's a cure I found on the internet.'

- 'Have you tried supplements?'

- 'Have you tried changing your diet?'

- 'I know someone who had ME, but now she runs marathons.'

I'm grateful that people take an interest and have taken the trouble to tell me about these things. The problem is, none of them are really relevant to me.

There are courses that suggest they can cure ME. Usually they're to do with positive thinking. It's possible that they may help some people cope with being ill, but they are not a cure. Neither are exercise or counselling. Exercise makes ME worse, even controlled 'graded' exercise (some doctors recommend exercise, but it's not a good idea). Counselling can help people cope with being ill, but it cannot make them better.

Right now, there is no cure for ME. Supplements and special diets may help certain symptoms, but they are unlikely to make a big difference.

I said earlier that it wasn't easy to explain about ME – it's not even easy to know what to call the illness. I'm going to tell you a bit more about that, because it might help explain why the person you know who runs marathons is different from me."

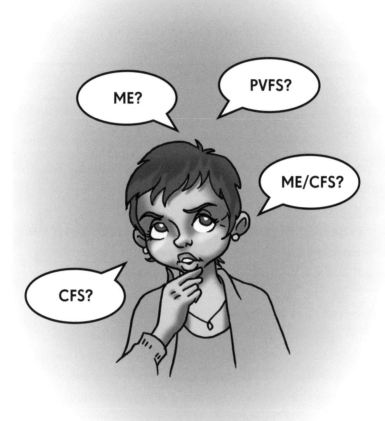

"What illness do we really have?"

Molly says:

"ME stands for myalgic encephalomyelitis (myalgic = muscle pain; encephalomyelitis = inflammation of the brain and spinal cord).

CFS stands for chronic fatigue syndrome (chronic = lasting a long time; fatigue = weariness after exertion).

Some people think these are different illnesses. They say that ME is a serious disease, but that CFS just means you have a mystery illness that includes fatigue.

Some doctors use the term CFS for everyone. A lot of patients don't like the name because it sounds like something that just makes you feel tired, but they have to use it because it's what their doctor says they have.

(To make things even more complicated, if a person's illness started with a virus – like mine did – their doctor might call it PVFS (post-viral fatigue syndrome) instead of ME or CFS.)

Because there aren't any tests that can say for sure whether you have ME or CFS, doctors decide what's wrong with you by ruling out other diseases then seeing how many symptoms you have that match a list of ME/CFS symptoms. The trouble is, different doctors use different lists (see p.60)! It makes things very difficult for PWME, and it also makes things difficult for doctors and scientists who do medical research, as it's not clear if everyone diagnosed with ME or CFS has the same illness.

So because of the different ways doctors have of deciding who has ME or CFS, it's entirely possible that two people with the same diagnosis have different illnesses – or that two people with different diagnoses have the same illness!"

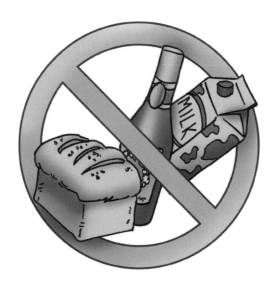

"Some people with ME have to
follow a restricted diet."

Ellie says:

"Mum's lucky, because there aren't really any foods that make her ill, but some PWME have to avoid sugar, or dairy products, or things like bread and pasta that have wheat in them. Some PWME feel sick a lot of the time so can only eat plain food. And some people who have ME really badly aren't able to eat proper food at all and have to be fed through a tube.

Mum does have to eat regularly, though – if she goes more than a few hours without eating, she starts to feel extra poorly and her body gets shaky. She keeps snacks by her bed in case she's not well enough to go downstairs to the kitchen to get something to eat, and she keeps cereal bars in her handbag for when she's out."

Molly says:

"I'm pleased food isn't a big problem for me – but I do sometimes struggle to eat healthily (and to feed my family healthy food) because I don't have the energy to prepare proper meals.

By the way, it's not just food that can cause problems for those who have ME. They may react badly to drugs (over-the-counter as well as prescribed medicines), to chemicals (anything from bathroom cleaner to hair dye), to alcohol (many PWME avoid it completely) and to anaesthetics or vaccinations."

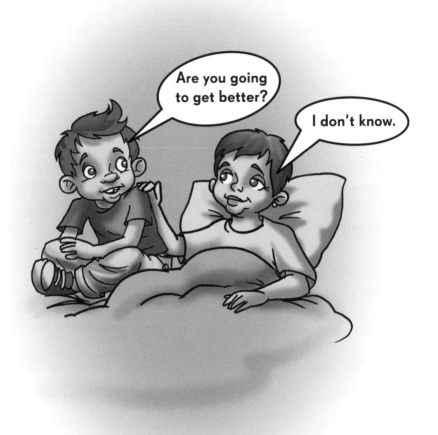

"The course of ME is unpredictable."

Eric says:

"A few years ago, Mum wasn't as ill as she is now, and she was able to do things like pick us up from school and take us to the park. Then she had a relapse – that means her illness got bad again – and she couldn't do those things any more. We've already explained that people with ME might have good days and bad days. Some people have good and bad *years*!

Some people's ME gets worse and worse. They might feel very, very ill and have to stay in bed all the time. We try to help Mum as much as possible because we don't want her to get that ill – but we know that if she *did* get worse, it wouldn't be our fault. Sometimes bad things like that just happen.

Mum says not to worry about her getting worse, though – it's just as likely that she'll get better again (she'll probably never get *completely* better, but anything would be good!). Perhaps her body will start healing itself, or doctors might discover some medicine that helps (some scientists already think they might have found some drugs that could help PWME – they just need to do lots of tests to make sure). Mum says if that happens we'll have a huge party!"

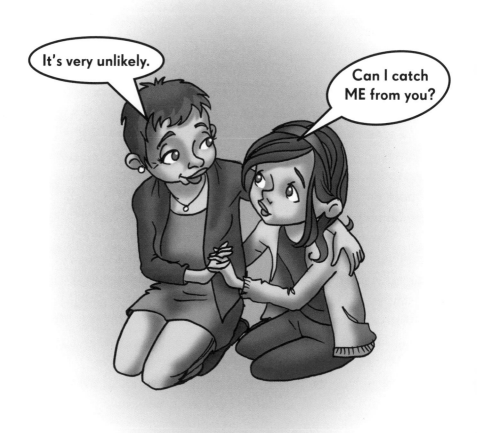

"Family and friends shouldn't worry
that they might get ill too

Ellie says:

"If I get a cold, usually everyone else in the family gets a cold because they catch it from me. I know not every disease can be passed on, but I've heard of families where more than one person has ME. Mum says, yes, that's true – but there are also thousands of families where only one person has ME.

Some people might be 'genetically susceptible' to ME. This means that something in their genes means they're more likely to get ME if certain conditions are met (for example, if they catch a virus when their body is already weak, perhaps from stress). In that case, someone who is related to a PWME might be *slightly* more likely to get ME than someone who isn't – but it *doesn't* mean they will definitely get ME.

Some doctors do think that ME is catching – but only at certain stages of the illness (for example, early on), or if it's a certain sort of ME (remember, we're still not sure if everyone who doctors say has ME or CFS has the same illness).

Don't forget that scientists still haven't found out exactly what causes ME, so a lot of this is guesswork – but there's really no need to worry."

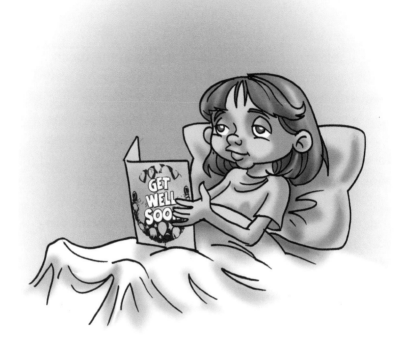

"Children can get ME too."

Eric and Ellie say:

"It's not just adults who get ME, children get it too. They don't get to do all the fun things we can do, such as play football or go to birthday parties. They might not be able to go to school. (You might think not going to school sounds great, but imagine never seeing your friends or learning any cool stuff.) Someone stuck at home with ME might not even have the energy to read a book or watch TV – that's got to be *really* boring.

Doctors say that children who have ME are more likely to recover than people who become ill when they're adults. And there's another thing that it's very important to remember – if someone is taking a long time getting better from a virus (like when our mum got glandular fever), the best thing they can do is rest *a lot*. If they do that, they might end up *not getting ME at all*!

So if one of your friends is ill, be understanding. Maybe you could send them a card or write them a letter (but say they don't have to send one back – it might be too much effort for them). Make sure they know it's OK to rest.

But if they don't get well – it's not their fault. They're still the same person, even if they can't do the same things they used to. Don't stop being their friend. They'll need friends more than ever."

How teachers can help

Molly says:

"Although Ellie and Eric aren't ill, my being ill affects them in all sorts of ways. Here are some of the things that it might help their teachers to be aware of:

- Children of PWME may have more responsibilities at home than other children. This means they may not have much time to spend on their homework, or they may be more tired at school. They may not be able to take part in extracurricular activities.

- We might not be able to attend school productions, or help with outings. We might not be able to contribute to bake sales or make costumes for dressing-up days. It might be difficult for us to help with homework projects. But none of this means we are not interested in our children or their progress at school!

- It's very easy for things to get forgotten or overlooked, both because ME causes memory problems and because lots of different people may be looking after the children over the course of a week. A 'Communications Book' where parents/ carers and teachers can keep each other 'in the loop' could prove useful.

- Perceived difference can be a cause of bullying. We hope that Eric and Ellie's teachers will look out for any signs of bullying due to them having an ill parent, such as teasing because their mum walks oddly or uses a wheelchair.

- There may be financial issues for a family with an ill parent."

List of acronyms

(Some of these terms are not used anywhere in this book, but are included as they are often found in ME/CFS literature.)

CCC: Canadian Consensus criteria

CFIDS: chronic fatigue and immune dysfunction syndrome

CFS: chronic fatigue syndrome

CNS: central nervous system

EDS: Ehlers–Danlos syndrome (a genetic connective-tissue condition, sometimes found alongside and sharing many symptoms with ME)

FM/FMS: fibromyalgia/fibromyalgia syndrome (colloquially known as "fibro" – a pain condition often found alongside ME)

ICC: International Consensus criteria

ME: myalgic encephalomyelitis

MS: multiple sclerosis (a neurological condition that may be misdiagnosed as ME, and vice versa)

OH: orthostatic hypotension (a condition causing low blood pressure upon standing, often found in ME sufferers)

PEM: post-exertional malaise

PENE: post-exertional neuroimmune exhaustion

POTS: postural orthostatic tachycardia syndrome (a condition causing increased heart rate upon standing, often found in PWME)

PVS/PVFS: post-viral syndrome/post-viral fatigue syndrome

PWCFS: person/people with CFS

PWME: person/people with ME

Facts and figures

- ME has been classified as a neurological illness by the World Health Organization since 1969.

- There are approximately 250,000 PWME in the UK, of which 25 per cent are classed as being severely affected.

- Approximately 10 per cent of PWME are children.

- Various criteria used for diagnosing ME or CFS include the London, Oxford, Fukuda, Canadian Consensus and International Consensus. (As of 2013, the International Consensus criteria are the most comprehensive.)

Recommended organisations and websites

UK

Invest in ME
PO Box 561
Eastleigh
Hampshire
SO50 0GQ
Phone: 02380 251719 or 07759 349743
Email: info@investinme.org
Website: http://investinme.org

NB A pdf of the International Consensus criteria, aka 'Myalgic Encephalomyelitis – Adult and Paediatric: International Consensus Primer for Medical Practitioners' can be found at this site.

Irish ME/CFS Association
PO Box 3075
Dublin 2
Phone: 01 235 0965
Email: info@irishmecfs.org
Website: www.irishmecfs.org

ME Research UK
The Gateway
North Methven Street
Perth
PH1 5PP
Phone: 01738 451234
Email: meruk@pkavs.org.uk
Website: www.meresearch.org.uk

The ME Association
7 Apollo Office Court
Radclive Road
Gawcott
Bucks
MK18 4DF
Phone: 01280 818964
Email: admin@meassociation.org.uk
Website: www.meassociation.org.uk

Tymes Trust (for children and young people with ME)
PO Box 4347
Stock
Ingatestone
CM4 9TE
Phone: 0845 003 9002
Email: jane.colby@tymestrust.org
Website: www.tymestrust.org

EUROPE

European ME Alliance
Website: www.euro-me.org

See website for details of member organisations in Belgium, Denmark, Germany, Holland, Ireland, Italy, Norway, Spain, Sweden, Switzerland and the UK.

CANADA

National ME/FM Action Network
512, 33 Banner Road
Nepean
ON K2H 8V7
Phone: 613 829 6667
Email: mefminfo@mefmaction.com
Website: www.mefmaction.com

US
OMI-MERIT (research)
2500 Hospital Drive, Bldg 2
Mountain View
CA 94040
Phone: 650 691 8633
Email: info@openmedicineinstitute.org
Website: http://openmedicineinstitute.org

AUSTRALIA
Alison Hunter Memorial Foundation
PO Box 6132
North Sydney
NSW 2059
Phone: 2 9958 6285
Email: chunter@ahmf.org
Website: www.ahmf.org

ME/CFS Australia
PO Box 120
Chapel Street
Prahan
VIC 3181
Phone: 03 9529 1344
Email: ceo@mecfs.org.au
Website: www.mecfs.org.au

Blank, for your notes

Blank, for your drawings